Essential Oils

Lose Weight, Improve Your Skin & Boost Your Happiness with Essential Oils

Table Of Contents

Introduction 1

Chapter 1: What Are Essential Oils? 4

Chapter 2: What Is Aromatherapy? 6

Chapter 3: The Different Ways To Use Essential Oils
.... 8

Chapter 4: The Healthy Benefits Of Using Essential
Oils 11

Essential Oils For Weight Loss 12

Essential Oils For Beautiful Skin 20

Essential Oils For Enhancing Your Mood 25

How Essential Oils Can Alter Your Mood 26

Chapter 5: Choosing The Best Oils And Storing Them
.... 28

Chapter 6: Safety Options While Using Essential Oils
.... 33

Conclusion 36

Free Bonus eBook Access: 15 Essential Oil Recipes
for Beauty Treatments 37

Introduction

We want to thank you and congratulate you for downloading the book, "Essential Oils: Lose Weight, Improve Your Skin & Boost Your Happiness with Essential Oils".

This book contains well-proven steps and strategies on how to make the most of essential oils. Essential oils have **many** great uses; this ranges from helping you shed weight, to improving the radiance of your skin and adding to the charming beauty and appeal of your face – and it doesn't just end there!

Aromatherapy, the art of using essential oils and aromatic plant extracts, is excellent for improving mental health by enhancing mood and boosting levels of happiness. These are **ancient practices** that have been around practically as long as humans have been interacting with the plant kingdom!

In this book, not only will we make you familiar with the different aspects and uses of essentials oils and aromatherapy, but also, we will deal with **important tips** on how to choose the best oils, ways of storing them efficiently and safe consumption of the oil.

This is an **ultimate guide** created to help you understand the vast applications of essential oils and how to use them to heal your mind, body and spirit.

Thanks for downloading this book, we hope you enjoy it!

The information herein is offered for informational purposes solely and is universal as so. The presentation of the information is without a contract or any guarantee assurance.

The trademarks that are used are without any consent, and the publication of the trademark is without permission or backing by the trademark owner. All trademarks and brands within this book are for clarifying purposes only and are the owned by the owners themselves, not affiliated with this document.

Chapter 1:
What Are Essential Oils?

Essential oils have been in use for many years now; more than 2000 years ago the distillation of essential oils began. This process was initially founded by alchemists, in a bid to aid in improved health and even longevity. Various forms of research indicate that back in the earlier times, a lot of simpler methods were used for extracting essential oils from plants, and it was subsequently used for several herbal preparations as well.

Essential oil is named so mainly because they contain the essence of the fragrant and therapeutic element of plants, however from the name we can even infer that it is essential to the health of our being since it is through the survival of plants and water that early humankind began to thrive!

In China, among the Chinese, essential oils are mainly used in the field of medicine and medicinal practice. It is believed that they were used as medicines for the Shen (spirit) as it is related to the spiritual essence which helps in healing the heart and mind.

According to the Ayurveda, essential oil is known to increase the flow of life force, known as Prana, as well as brightening mental luminosity. It is further believed that essential oils aid in improving the immune system and overall physical/mental vitality.

There are countless numbers of oils with many benefits, and the healing properties of their aromas are limitless. This is why it is often considered to be impossible to tap into all the possible uses of essential oils.

Essential oil is also believed to be the quintessential oil. According to Aristotle, matter is mainly made of four different elements, namely fire, air, earth and water. A fifth element was later added which was known as quintessence, which is considered to be the life force.

The process used to extract oil from plants is mainly via distillation, however there are plenty of other methods which can be used and this includes:

- Solvent extraction

- Resin tapping

- Cold pressing

- Expression

- Absolute oil extraction

These techniques vary based on their application in the world. Essential oil extractions are used in a number of different industrial areas such as perfumes, natural food flavoring, soaps, cosmetics, beauty products, and even incense and natural home-cleaning solutions.

Now, let us venture deep into the world of essential oils to help you get an even clearer idea of how essential oils can be used, bought and stored!

Chapter 2:
What Is Aromatherapy?

Aromatherapy is mainly a form of alternative medicine which makes use of essential oils and plenty of other aromatic plants for the sake of improving the physical health of a person and their mood.

Many people believe that this method of treatment is considered to be unscientific, yet there isn't concrete evidence to prove this, although there have been efforts in the recent past to add some evidence to it.

Aromatherapy refers to the art of utilizing the aromatic essence present in the plant by extracting them naturally to create the right balance and harmony in your body, mind and spirit.

The History

It was in the 1920s that the term aromatherapy was coined. However, using essential oils for improving human health can be traced back to thousands of years ago.

According to historical records, it is believed that it was the Ancient Egyptians who first invented the distillation equipment which is used for aromatherapy. They started using the oils extracted from herbs in different rituals and even in perfumes and cosmetics.

Later, a French chemist by the name of Rene-Maurice Gatterfosse gave birth to the term 'Aromatherapy'. He once experienced an extremely painful burn which led him to plunge his burned hand in a nearby vat of lavender oil, which was seen merely as a industrial solution. He was astonished as he saw how quickly he recovered from his burns!

He went on to study the many details and applications of these oils and became one of the world's renowned Aromatherapists. He published the book "Gattefosse's Aromatherapy" which contains some of the earliest clinical findings of essential oils. He coined the word, "Aromatherapie" which inferred the therapeutic use of aromatic substances which can be used in a holistic manner for healing.

To make things even more clear, let us present a few quotes by some eminent Aromatherapists:

"Aromatherapy is a caring, hands-on therapy which seeks to induce relaxation, to increase energy, to reduce the effects of stress and to restore lost balance to mind, body and soul." -**Robert Tisserand**

"Aromatherapy is the skilled and controlled use of essential oils for physical and emotional health and well-being." - **Valerie Cooksley**

"It is a natural, non-invasive modality designed to affect the whole person, not just the symptom or disease and to assist the body's natural ability to balance, regulate, heal and maintain itself by the correct use of essential oils." - **Jade Shutes**

So, with this clear understanding of what aromatherapy is and some of its rich history, we will proceed to learning their various uses and applications.

Chapter 3:
The Different Ways To Use
Essential Oils

It is essential for one to know that essential oils have a varied number of uses and applications, which we will list here in detail.

1. Aerial Diffusion

This is mainly used to make the oil evaporate and blend with the air. The aim of this application is give the air the oil's specific fragrance and therapeutic value.

We all love a sweet aroma which can make the whole environment pleasant and ebullient. When using essential oil diffusers, it creates a great ambiance. The diffusers make use of the vibration of water molecules for dispensing the essential oil into the air.

This is applicable at homes, offices and even classrooms as the scent of these oils could help you to stay focused and alert.

2. Topical Applications

You can apply the aromatic oil directly on your skin; this can be during massage, baths, and even for cosmetic purposes.

While topical use is common and well-practiced, it is important to check the particular oil you wish to apply and its properties. While most oils do not produce side effects, some are more concentrated and powerful than others and can cause irritation for sensitive skin. It is important to be aware!

3. Direct Inhalation

In this form, the person makes it a point to breathe the essential oil directly. This aids in the treatment of respiratory infections and even decongestion. It helps one to feel calm, uplifted and centered. The two forms of direct inhalation are:

Direct bottle inhalation

Direct bottle inhalation refers to the method of sniffing or inhaling the essential oil directly from the bottle. This particular form of inhalation finds its use predominantly for helping people deal with emotional and stress-related problems.

Direct palm inhalation

Direct palm inhalation refers to the method of sniffing or inhaling the essential oil directly from the palms of your hand. This particular form of inhalation finds its use predominantly for helping people deal with respiratory and breathing problems.

Direct inhalation techniques are a fast and effective way to immediately aid in calming down a person, especially those who are suffering from anxiety issues, emotional distress and various problems relating to the nervous system.

4. Smelling Salts

In this form, we create a synergy of 20-30 drops, making use of 2 to 5 different essential oils. You should place the mix in a small 10ml bottle. When you have placed the oil mix in the bottle, fill the rest of it with fine or coarse sea salts. Place these enhanced salts in your bathtub, or just leave the bottle open next to you to absorb the various benefits of your chosen oil mix.

5. Absorption through cloth or cotton balls

You can place a few drops of essential oil or on a cloth or cotton ball. Now, hold the cloth/cotton in your palm and inhale deeply through your nose. This use is excellent because the absorption of the cloth/cotton allows for more surface area to be covered and more of the oil will be exposed.

Be creative! There are lots of ways to use the oils you choose, and there is so much to be gained! You can use any of these methods to instantly relieve stress, uplift mood, support regular breathing, reduce nasal congestion, improve hormonal balance, improve emotional stability, and much more!

Chapter 4:
The Healthy Benefits Of Using Essential Oils

Congratulations!

We are so happy to have people read this in an effort to change their life in a healthy and natural way – and by reading this book you are definitely coming closer to your positive transformation!

Change never comes in a day, especially when we are talking about the human body which is a marvel in itself. To attain the desired state of health which you have in mind, you will need to work hard. It is not only about getting into shape, but it is more about choosing a healthier lifestyle. Essential oils can help you not only to regulate physical health, but also to come closer to nature by understanding your body.

In today's hectic world, it becomes pretty tough to know your own body. When we are busy with everyday modern tasks, we begin to slowly disconnect from, and start to become alien to ourselves. It is important to break this pattern and be closer to the gifts of mother earth. Hopefully, through this guide, you may gain more awareness of the significant change that essential oils can bring to your life.

When we inhale our desired essence, it stays with us throughout the day. Our mind can register a fragrance the same way we remember words over breakfast or an old memory from years ago. Often, a perfume reminds us of a loved one and an aroma of a delicious meal takes us back to those good childhood days. Scents can stimulate your mind in many ways, and can even take you back to your past.

What makes essential oils so beneficial are the particles that are infused in them, which vary based on the extraction of various parts of flowers, barks, resins, roots, and other organics plants. It has been discovered that the Ancient Egyptians used to make essential oils by soaking various natural ingredients in a carrier/host oil and further filtering the oil with the help of a linen bag. We have certainly come a long way since then; still the central mechanism is still the same for organically creating essential oils.

Essential oils contain the kind of fragrance that can not only help you sleep or relax your senses, but can also provide substantial results to your body, like balancing your digestive system, improving your skin, and so much more that elevates their importance of a pleasant smell. They are in use for more than thousands of years, dating back to our early ancestors. Various cultures and civilizations around the world have been found using essential oils for health and medical purposes for years – from aromatherapy to beauty treatments to industrial applications and much more.

Please note: It is strongly advised to seek professional guidance before using any essential oils internally or topically, especially without first diluting the oil. Some oils can be very concentrated, and not all oils are created with equal potency. People have different levels of tolerance and sensitivity as well, so please use caution and seek professional guidance before use. More information on safety can be found in Chapter 6.

Essential Oils For Weight Loss

One of the major benefits of using essential oils is to regulate weight. There have been multiple studies done by various academicians and universities in the past about the significance of essential oils and how their usage can help an individual to lose weight. For instance, just the scent of lemon or grapefruit oil can trigger your body to burn fat and slow weight gain.

Using essential oils will not only help you to lose weight, but also to maintain a healthy lifestyle and target weight on a constant basis. There are various kinds of essential oils that can help you lose weight. They are explained below as every kind of essential oil has its own unique characteristics that can help you in different ways.

1. **Grapefruit Oil**

   Grapefruit oil is probably the most extensively used type of essential oil for weight loss. It is extracted from the ingredients of the grapefruit peel that contain a large amount of D-limonene. It is a very crucial compound as it works wonders to maintain the metabolic activities in your body. It goes to your lymphatic glands and drains them to achieve a healthy and clean flow. Grapefruit can activate different enzymes in your body that can end up breaking down body fat.

   You can always mix grapefruit oil with other essential oils to amplify its results. For example, when grapefruit oil is mixed with patchouli oil, it can lower your feelings of hunger. It can also help in the retention of water in your body. Apart from physical comfort, it can help you feel relaxed and fight against stress and tension. If you know someone who is suffering from overeating or depression, you should suggest that they use this amazing essential oil.

   Applying grapefruit oil is very easy. You can simply diffuse a few drops of it near your personal space –

whether it is your office or your home. You can massage it on your chest or wrist, or add a small drop of it to your water to give it a fresh flavor. Try massaging some on your wrist when you are craving some food and see the incredible results!

2. **Ginger Oil**

The second most significant essential oil that is used to regulate weight is ginger oil. It helps drastically to reduce cravings for sugar and decreases the inflammation in the body. While diet and exercise is essential to cutting the excess fat out of your body, it is of high significance that you reduce inflammation and take care of your digestive system as well.

The compound that is responsible for fighting against body weight, found in ginger is known as 'gingerol'. It can help to escalate the level of vitamin and mineral absorption in your body, as well as decrease the intestinal inflammation in your system, side-effect free. The absorption of all the good vitamins and minerals will help you strengthen your immune system and let you get prepared for the weight loss training. They will escalate the energy of your cells and give you the much-needed will to walk that extra mile to burn those unwanted calories.

Gingerol is extracted from the active part of the ginger root, making it extremely potent. We recommend that instead of applying ginger oil in a concentrated form, first dilute it a little to neutralize its strong essence. Apply the diluted form of the oil on your abdomen. In case if you are feeling uneasy, take a cotton ball or a tissue and put a drop of ginger oil on it. Afterward, rub the cotton ball or tissue on your wrists or abdomen for immediate comfort.

According to the recent studies on ginger oil, it has been found that gingerol has significant amounts of antioxidants, making the oil a true essential for every individual who would like to sustain the path of health. The research was carried out on mice, and after a few days of being treated with ginger oil, the enzyme levels in their body increased and their blood flow became better. We suggest that you treat your body with some ginger essential oil for at least a month to see the substantial changes in your health.

3. **Cinnamon Oil**

Widely known for its aroma and mesmerizing essence, cinnamon oil is also extensively used to cut the extra weight from our body. There have been a lot of studies that were done that clearly depicted the benefits of cinnamon oil. Studies show that cinnamon oil helps to retain the Glucose Tolerance Factor (GTF) in the body, which is important for people who are suffering from diabetes. Cinnamon oil, like ginger oil, helps those with diabetes control their cravings for sugar while regulating the level of glucose in their system.

Besides the above-stated benefits, cinnamon oil balances blood pressure in the long term; helping one to achieve their weight loss target. It has been scientifically observed that an unstable level of blood pressure causes trouble to the heart, and can also result in overeating, weight gain, and energy loss. One of the best ways of using cinnamon oil is to apply a little on grains or vegetables. It will impart a sweet and desirable essence to the food. You can also add it to your everyday favorites like tea, oats, fruits, or smoothies. Since cinnamon has a favorable smell that everyone loves, you can simply pour few drops on your pillow or leave an open bottle in your office to inhale its sweet essence to have a healthy mind during work.

Besides weight loss, it also strengthens your immune system, neutralizes your appetite, and increases your metabolism. An improved metabolic system will end up making you slimmer by speeding up the digestive process. To attain overall balance in your body, it can aid in increasing blood circulation and improving the digestive system. It increases libido and fights against the toxins present in your body gently with time. A daily consumption of cinnamon oil for at least a month certainly show you obvious and visible changes in your body.

4. **Peppermint Oil**

This might come as a surprise, but peppermint oil has been extensively used for years to neutralize appetite and decrease cravings for hunger. It is also widely used to increase one's stamina before exercise. Simply smell it before hitting the gym and see the difference in your long workout sessions.

It is an excellent choice to fight against any growing digestion issues. Apart from digestion, the oil helps an individual stimulate their mind and disconnect from stress or any unwanted tension. It is often used to treat Candida, which is tightly related to weight gain.

An upset stomach is often related to poor eating habits or impulsive cravings, which can cause one to make poor dietary choices. With an intake of a few drops of peppermint oil, you can get rid of an upset stomach and slow down cravings, giving you time to prepare a healthy meal instead of impulsive snacking. It will give you an elevated feeling of satisfaction after eating, so you won't have frequent cravings for food. It will also help your body derive more energy from the food so that you stay healthy and fit all day long.

There are many ways of applying peppermint oil. One way is to pour a few drops of the oil on a cotton ball and gradually inhale its vapors. This should be done before you consume anything so that you have a satisfying meal and won't end up overeating. If you are aiming to reduce the intake of food substantially, then try adding just a few small drops of it in a glass of water and drinking it before a meal for a healthy appetite. If you want to kick start your day with full energy, then add a few drops of peppermint oil to a hot bath and have an amazing experience! The essence of this oil will stay with you throughout the day, making you feel brand new!

5. Lemon Oil

Lemon oil has a strong and fresh essence that can make you maintain your very best mood all day long, with numerous health benefits. It is widely known that lemon oil detoxifies our body and keeps our energy high for the day. The citric element which is present in lemon oil diminishes the parasites present in our intestines, helping us clean up our digestive tract.

Often toxins find their place in various fat cells in our body. Intake of lemon oil will clean your body and prevent these toxins from being stored. You already know the importance of grapefruit oil and how it fights against weight gain; just like grapefruit oil, lemon oil also consists of D-limonene that fights against fat cells and helps promote a clean and healthy body. It supplies a wide range of vitamins and minerals to your body that helps to keep a balance of your metabolic rate. One of the main ingredients that are present in lemon oil is vitamin C, which not only fights against infection and parasites in your intestines, but also helps you preserve energy and lose weight in a healthy manner.

Since lemon oil has a fresh and desirable flavor, it can be used in numerous ways. From infusing a few drops on your clothes and bed, to drinking it with hot water. A regular intake of lemon oil can create wonders in your life!

6. Sandalwood Oil

Calm, soothing, and delightful, Sandalwood oil is one of those widely used essential oils that are desired by everyone for its restful and relaxing essence. It is most commonly used by people who are suffering from stress related eating. If you are among the group of many people who tends to eat whenever they are stressed, then you should start using sandalwood oil. Today, stress eating is one of the primary reasons behind obesity and is done by thousands of people all over the globe.

Sandalwood oil has a calm and relaxing aura that will allow your mind to wind down. The regular intake of this essential oil might even influence a change of perspective towards your life. It can help you fight against pessimism and make room for optimistic feelings to flow. You will see the change in your behavior that will stop you from the amount of undesirable emotional eating. After a few weeks of inhaling its soothing essence, you will come to realize that you don't need to eat more to deal with the amount of ongoing tension in your life.

7. Bergamot Oil

A tropical plant and one of the most widely used citrus fruits – Bergamot has always been associated with good health and will for thousands of years to come. It is often consumed by people who have a bad digestive system as it can help to stimulate the liver and spleen. If you know someone who is going through a bad phase or is depressed, then start applying a few drops of bergamot oil to their surroundings to uplift their spirit. If you have a tendency to overeat, then apply a little bergamot oil before any meal to avoid the chances of eating more than you really need to feel satisfied.

The most talked about, and well-researched ingredient that is found in bergamot oil is polyphenols. It is the same compound that is found in green tea that helps our body to burn fat and stops our craving for sugar. The essence of bergamot oil can be used to prepare a hot bath or can be used the old fashion way – by rubbing it against your wrists.

Essential Oils For Beautiful Skin

Essential oils are not only used to get one in their best shape, but they are also extensively used to attain flawless skin. If you are going through any skin related ailment, then you must make use of this essential oil. We have come up with a comprehensive list of various essential oils that can help you to achieve beautiful, glowing, and flawless skin – side effect free!

1. **Helichrysum Oil**

   This vibrant yellow flower has some vital elements that are used by several skin care and cosmetic products. It has been observed that Helichrysum oil can drastically reduce the wrinkles of your skin and be a great aid to multiply the natural collagen count of your skin, leading to a natural and a toned finish. If you have a scar, a wounded tissue, or any bruise on your skin, then treat it with Helichrysum oil and see it healing fast in time. The best way to apply Helichrysum oil is by blending it with either rose infused oil or in other carriers like jojoba oil or rosehip seed oil for best results.

2. **Carrot Seed Oil**

   Rejuvenate your skin like never before with some carrot seed oil, and see your skin begin to glow! It can help you achieve an even tone of your skin while reducing the amount of scars and other aging spots that may be visible.

   Carrot seed oil constitutes an essential ingredient to produce various facial cosmetic products, especially moisturizers. Apply a few drops of this oil to attain healthy and well-nourished skin. If you are planning to create a home-made beauty product, then be sure apply a little carrot seed oil to your mixture. Queen Anne's lace, which is known as wild carrot seed oil, is considered a universal skin treatment solution due to its anti-aging effect.

3. Rose Oil

If you have a dry and aging skin, then you must try rose essential oil. Rose oil has some anti-inflammatory and antimicrobial properties present which can cause a therapeutic and healing effect on your body and skin. These characteristics of the rose essential oil help to give your skin a refined tone and texture. If you know someone who is suffering from skin conditions like dermatitis or psoriasis, then recommend them to apply rose essential oil, as it can significantly help their condition.

Since Rose oil has a desirable fragrance, a lot of people simply inhale it to have a calm and soothed mood. It has been found that simply inhaling the oil can slow extra water loss from your skin, letting it maintain its natural charm and glow. It has a relaxing fragrance that inhibits the development of the hormone 'cortisol' in your body, which is responsible for causing stress. It is widely known that a stress-free individual will always have flawless skin and a healthy attitude.

4. Frankincense Oil

Known to have anti-inflammatory and antibacterial properties, it works wonders for your skin, especially if your skin is acne-prone. Frankincense oil is known to be a natural toner as it evens the skin tone and diminishes various pores and black spots on the skin. It increases the growth of new cells and protects the existing cells from tearing, promoting smooth skin. If you would like to reduce scars, wrinkles and tighten your skin, then Frankincense oil is your best treatment.

5. Tea Tree Oil

Tea tree oil has antibacterial properties that diminishes the occurrence of any acne causing bacteria on your skin. It not only helps you to attain smooth and flawless skin, but also promotes healthy nails and cuticles. It is used to strengthen the bond of cells and to promote the growth of new cells so that you have fresh and glowing skin consistently. Mix it with your preferred ointment or moisturizer for best results.

6. Geranium Oil

The moment you think you are going to have an acne breakout, make use of geranium essential oil to get the best and immediate results. It is proven that geranium oil works well to tighten the skin and to increase the skin's elasticity, which reduces the occurrence of wrinkles to a great extent. It helps to regulate blood flow so that all your skin parts are hydrated and full of blood supply. Apply some geranium oil to your bruises and scars and say goodbye to all skin related problems.

7. Neroli Oil

If you have oily or sensitive skin, then you must apply neroli essential oil provide an even tone skin with fine lining. It will also rejuvenate the skin cells, making you look younger every day. It has a natural compound, known as Citral, which is responsible for skin regeneration. Since the oil has prominent skin regeneration properties, it makes it easier for you to heal scars, bruises, and most significantly, stretch marks.

If you are worried that your skin is producing a lot of oil, causing you to lose essential nutrients, then you must apply neroli oil to the oily area. It will shrink your pores so that your skin will be restricted and excrete less oil, but won't be dry as a result.

8. Leleshwa Oil

Leleshwa essential oil is popularly known to have purifying characteristics as it can renew and rejuvenate the skin cells. Also, if you are facing hair fall or problems related to your nails, then Leleshwa oil would be of great help to you. When you are using Leleshwa oil, you must take caution as it is a potent oil and should always be mixed with another kind of carrier oil. Simply add it to your lotion or body oil before applying it on your skin or nails.

If you are using it on your hair, then add it to your normal shampoo to provide nutritive benefits to your hair and scalp. If your skin has any imperfections such as a scar or bruise, then treat it with some Leleshwa oil to get improved results.

9. Ylang Ylang Oil

Extracted from the exotic flower, ylang-ylang oil is known all over the world for its benefits. It is one of the most preferred essential oils used to provide perfection to your skin while imparting its soothing scent. The best thing about ylang-ylang oil is that it suits every skin type. If you have oily skin, then applying this oil will minimize breakouts and reduce the production of oil.

Similarly, if you have dry skin, then regular usage of ylang-ylang oil will improve the elasticity of your skin and smooth out all the fine lines. Trusted for centuries, this essential oil will help you to attain beautiful and youthful skin on a regular basis. A tonic for the entire human body, it also helps to regenerate hair and reduce their fall after regular use.

10. Myrrh Oil

A must-have anti-aging product, Myrrh oil has powerful anti-inflammatory characteristics that not only reduce the occurrences of wrinkles and lines on your skin, but will also increase its elasticity and firmness. Healing sun damage and wrinkles, it will help you maintain your natural glow all day long.

11. Patchouli Oil

Last, but not least, an essential oil that every individual should have in their cabinet – Patchouli oil has several antifungal, antibacterial, and antiseptic properties that make it a household essential. Not only does it help to fight against wrinkles, it is also considered as a cure for serious skin-related diseases like dermatitis, eczema, psoriasis, and more. If you have acne-prone skin, then apply Patchouli oil regularly to see the change in your skin.

Patchouli has a sweet and desirable fragrance, which makes it one of the prime ingredients to manufacture perfumes and scented cosmetic products. If your nails are getting yellowed or cracked, then mix a few drops of Patchouli oil with a carrier oil and apply it to your nails to get instant results. Used by individuals for years, it is highly effective to maintain a natural and youthful glow your skin.

Essential Oils For Enhancing Your Mood

When you know that essential oils can not only make you shed weight but can also better your skin and hair, it becomes important to explore whether there are other useful applications of it.

Scent is one of the most powerful natural characteristics as it can change our mood drastically. The sense of smell is the most underrated sense of the human body, and it is time that you realize the potential power of a good fragrance.

A particular fragrance can sometimes work wonders on the mind and can take one to exotic places they have never been before. There is a reason why we humans are fond of perfumes and fragrances; they invoke memories or a visual scene, and the oil's essence has the power to change our emotions.

Essential oils have been used as a mood enhancer for centuries. With their different aromas and nature, different kinds of oils have their unique impact on our mind and body. Alter the aroma of your living space and be elated with the essential oil of your choice.

We already know that essential oils have various benefits related to aromatherapy, which has altered the lives of many people all over the world. When you feel sad, depressed, or tense, then you should use aromatherapy to set the perfect mood around you, making you feel restored and content. Don't wait any longer and start experimenting with various fragrances to find your favorite!

How Essential Oils Can Alter Your Mood

Before we learn the different kinds of essential oils that can make us happier, it is important to know how they work to change your mind and elevate the senses.

1. They are entirely made up of natural ingredients. No undesirable additives, synthetics, or cheap alcohols are used to create their fragrance. Pure and unadulterated, they come from the core of mother earth to impart a natural essence around you.

2. Their scent hits various neurons of the brain and enhances human sense, which not only elevates one's mood, but also imparts a positive nature to an individual. They also affect various hormonal changes and productions in the body in such a way that allows you to feel calm and good.

3. Scientifically speaking, consider essential oils as the extraction of plant matter, which contains the most vital compounds of the plant. When these compounds are transferred to your brain, they rapidly trigger the mind to send a powerful, yet calming and peaceful signal to the rest of the body. This creates feelings of balance, stability and heightened awareness.

4. They have the positive energy of mother earth that inspires you to lead a happy and content life. They have

no negative side-effects, which makes them so useful and important.

Lavender, sage, and bergamot essential oils are already widely known to stimulate your mind and enhance your mood. We have selected a few other essential oils that work great as a mood enhancer below:

- Clary sage's Oil

- Geranium Oil

- Grapefruit Oil

- Lemon Oil

- Neroli Oil

- Chamomile Oil

- Rose Oil

- Sandalwood Oil

- Sweet Orange Oil

- Cinnamon Bark Oil

Chapter 5:
Choosing The Best Oils And Storing Them

There are many companies that market essential oils and it is important to sort out the best ones among them. This can be done by looking for the ones which are likely to offer you the best quality at the right price. Here we will help you to learn some top tricks and details which will turn out to be handy in making the right selection.

Purity

This has to be the top factor in determining the oil to choose. When shopping for essential oils that can improve your health, you do not want to purchase impure or non-therapeutic grade oil.

While most companies are likely to use the word 'pure' when marketing their oil, using the word 'pure' doesn't necessarily make it pure.

Moreover, in the US, there is no legal meaning of this word. This is why before you decide to purchase a specific essential oil, you should make it a point to research thoroughly about the brand. This will give you a clear idea as to what grade and quality the oil is.

Synthetic Fragrances

There are a few oils that are exclusively available in the form of synthetic fragrances. Some of these names include

- Gardenia

- Frangipani

- Honeysuckle

- Linden

We wouldn't recommend synthetic oils because they might not impart the same benefits which are found in natural therapeutic oils. Of course, the smell and healing properties of natural oil and synthetic fragrances are going to differ a great deal. If you find that a whole line of essential oils are priced nearly the same, it is likely that the oil is synthetic.

Adulteration

This is yet another common problem you need to be wary of. There are a few oils which tend to be excessively adulterated because they are usually very expensive. To cut down costs, some manufacturers tend to mix cheap and inferior filler oils with the more expensive oil they are selling. This is common with oils like rose and sandalwood.

Of course, using adulterated oil is going to greatly diminish its benefit and strength, and this is why it is important to sort between mixed oil and pure oil while shopping.

Birch is one of the common essential oils which is often substituted with wintergreen and the latter is inexpensive but has quite similar characteristics. Inspect thoroughly and check the details to ensure that the essential oil that you are buying is pure and raw rather than mixed with inferior oils.

Grades

There are a lot of sellers who tend to sell low grade oil. Check the details of the seller and brand, and closely inspect them to ensure that the extraction is pure and potent.

The Supply Chain

When it comes to essential oils, you are likely to find many middlemen in the chain. Ideally, you should try to find suppliers from whom you can directly purchase the oil. When the oil is passed through a number of hands, say three or four, each step may add some adulteration and price inflation. In the end, the essential oil which you will get will not just be overpriced, but also adulterated and lacking quality.

There are so many suppliers and brands out there, that the best option would be to find a trustworthy essential oil distiller. This is the best way to guarantee the lowest price for the highest grade of oil

Perfume Oils

Never make a mistake of buying perfume oils with the thought that they are the same as essential oils. Perfume oils lack the therapeutic benefits which the essential oils have to offer.

Knowledge Base

When you are looking to expand your use of essential oils even further than this book, there is so much information out there! Aroma Web has a lot of information and even safety tips which come in very handy. It is advised that you read all the details about the safety actions to be taken when using essential oil.

The Right Comparison

One common mistake which a lot of people make is that they compare totally unrelated essential oils because of how similar they can be in name.

There are a lot of sub-varieties of each plant. The oils which are derived from these sub-varieties can be extremely different; they will have their own unique healing properties.

When you pay close heed to the botanical name of the oils, you will be able to trace how related the oils are and if they have been derived from the same plant.

The Source

We advise you to note the country where the essential oil you intend to buy has originated. Ideally, sellers should readily offer you the botanical name of the oil along with its country of origin. Make a point to check if the oils offered are ethically farmed, organic or wild-crafted. These minor details play a crucial role when trying to determine the best quality.

Where to Buy?

While it is common that a lot of people purchase essential oils at craft shows, fairs, and vendors, it is not considered the best place to buy. There are vendors who know that the buyers will have no access to contact them later and this makes them fearless – they may end up selling you inferior and low quality oil.

This is not to say that we are completely against buying at fairs; there could surely be some reputable and established sellers out there. However, unless you are a pro at buying essential oils and know how to separate one from the other, there is no need to rush in the buying process. If you are not sure about the seller, you should refrain from purchasing from them.

Storage Tips

You should make it a point to store the oils in dark glasses; this prevents damage from light. They can be either amber or cobalt blue color. The oil should always be stored in a room temperature and dark place, so a closed cabinet or drawer is ideal.

These are the simple yet effective precautionary measures which will help you prolong the life of your essential oil collection. Now, we will be heading to next chapter where we will discuss the safety aspect.

Chapter 6:
Safety Options While Using Essential Oils

The use of essential oils are considered to be quite harmless if used safely and applied correctly. However, the selection of essential oils is fairly huge and varied, and there are a large number of different oils out there which are still being researched and their potential dangers are poorly known.

Here are some of the safety points which you should implement for the sake of ensuring that your use of essential oils does not cause you any problems:

- Never use essential oils internally until a professional practitioner has guided you or asked you to do so.

- When you are opting for the topical application of an essential oil, you need to dilute it by using a carrier oil as this will ensure that even though it is in a concentrated form, it won't harm your skin.

- If you are going out and will be exposed to UV rays, it is advised not to expose your body to citrus oil because this may intensify the effect of the sun.

- Always make sure to keep your oil away from the reach of the children.

- You should make sure that you do not let the oil come in close contact with your mucous membranes or your eyes.

- If you know someone who has a serious medical ailment, do not use an essential oil on them without the right advice or guidance from a medical practitioner.

- Always make it a point to use pure essential oils and avoid the use of synthetic fragrances.

- When you are storing your oils, follow our tips on storage as it will help in ensuring that the oils will last long and won't degrade quickly.

One important tip to keep in mind is in regards to the biocompatible levels of the ingestion of essential oil. To make things clear, let us use the example of oregano oil. Oregano oil is a popular choice, and known to be used for internal consumption as well as for its therapeutic benefits. However, it is often seen that due to internal consumption of oregano oil, people sometimes experience gastric issues as it can lead to hyperacidity. If you end up having an accidental over-ingestion of an essential oil, you should make it a point to get instantly in touch with your local poison center.

There are a few oils like lavender that are known to be completely safe for use and are devoid of any kinds of problems. However even so, some people may develop an allergic response. This is why you are advised to be cautious when using essential oils.

Skin reactivity

Many people have sensitive skin, and this makes it hard for them to carelessly use essential oils. If your skin is sensitive, it is important to be careful. The main problems arise from mixing synthetic aromatic chemicals with essential oils. These synthetic chemicals can be reactive, and it can cause damage to the skin.

Before applying large amounts of an oil solution to your skin, you should start with patch testing. Patch testing is the process wherein only a small area of your skin is tested with the diluted oil before applying the oil to a larger area.

Photo-toxicity

There are a few essential oils that are known to increase your sensitivity to sunlight when you use them on your body. They can be harmful if they are not diluted well.

Irritation

There are a few oils which are known to have a strong irritant nature. These oils include garlic, onion, mustard and horseradish. They are typically know to be mildly irritating, but if you have sensitive skin, it can lead to more serious issues. This is why you need to steer clear of irritating oils when you have skin sensitivity issues.

Conclusion

Thank you again for downloading this book!

I hope were able to help you to understand the various details about essential oils, and have made you familiar with all the benefits they can bring. There are so many oils out there, with so many healing properties – its truly amazing! Nature has all the answers out there, and we do not need synthetic drugs to regulate our mood, weight and well-being.

We made it a point to discuss both the positive and potentially dangerous aspects of essential oils so that you could accurately understand everything without any biases. Essential oils can greatly benefit your health, but as everything in life – balance is the key. Be sure to take caution in how you use these oils, as they can be very powerful in whichever way you use them.

Make it a point to go through the book as many times as needed and get familiar with all the varied ways by which you can use essential oils to improve your physical health, mental health and spiritual connection.

Their benefits are endless!

Free Bonus eBook Access:
15 Essential Oil Recipes for Beauty Treatments

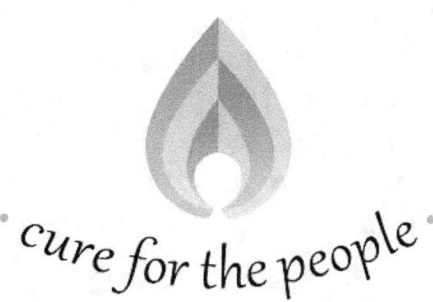

cure for the people

We really hope you enjoyed reading this book, and we want you to know that **we care about our community and the people in it**. That's why we began our collective called 'Cure For The People'. We love to publish lots of different content on various subjects from health to self-help, and much more. We want to open the minds and hearts of our readers, to spread awareness on important topics and have a good time doing it! However, we cannot do what we love to do... without you! Community is the most important part of this movement, and **we want you** to be a part of it!

We would love for you to interact with us and other like-minded individuals on our social media pages, as well as read more great articles and blogs on various related topics, and even get **free chapters from our other books** – all to be found on our website:

www.cure4people.com

You can also find more of our books and video trailers on Amazon which we know **you will LOVE**, by simply visiting our Amazon Author page:

www.amazon.com/author/cure4people

And one last, final thing...

Like we said earlier, community is the most important element required to continue spreading awesome life-changing information to the world – and so if we want people to discover and learn, we need people to trust us and our books! If you could be so kind and helpful, could you please leave us an **honest review** on our Amazon page for this book? We made it super easy and provided the link right here:

www.amazon.com/review/create-review

We give you our big thanks in advance for this super-awesome favor!

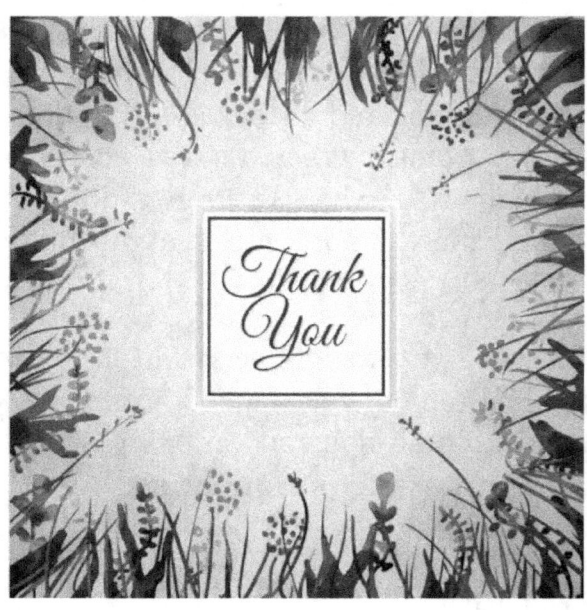

As a big 'THANK YOU' we have written a free bonus eBook, *just for you.* It's an eBook that has no availability or access anywhere but right here. As an even bigger bonus, when you download the free book, you will be subscribed to our newsletter which will continue to provide you **additional valuable content** on this particular subject. We want to continue supporting our readers by engaging with them after they read our books and this is the perfect way to stay connected.

So.. for the moment we have all been waiting for... We present to you... your free bonus ebook:

"15 Essential Oil Recipes for Beauty Treatments"

www.cure4people.com/essential-oils-bonus-486

We hope you enjoy this free content, and we wish to continue our relationship through our newsletter, social media channels, website and blog.

Best Wishes from the Cure For The People family!